SLEEP LIKE A
WINNER!
TREATMENT OF INSOMNIA

—— A 6-WEEK PROGRAM TO HELP YOU SLEEP WELL ——

ABDUL QADIR, MD

ISBN: 978-1-7368357-0-8

ACKNOWLEDGMENT

This book is dedicated to my family members who have helped me throughout the journey of my career and this book.

Thanks to my mother who raised us as a single mom.

Thanks to my maternal uncles who supported us during our difficult childhood.

Thanks to my brother Ali who was not only a fatherly figure for me but also a great friend

I would also like to thank the love of my life, my wife Bushra, who has always supported me in my career.

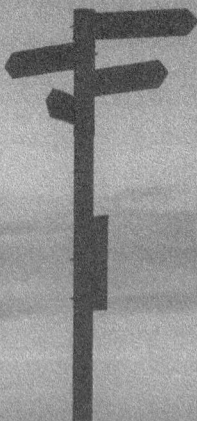

Be the change you wish to see in the world.

\- Gandhi

TABLE OF CONTENTS

ABOUT THE AUTHOR

Dr Abdul Qadir is a Board-Certified Psychiatrist in the State of California. He has worked extensively with people who suffer from Sleep Disorder and Stress Related problems. He has treated many clients who are going through Insomnia.

He works in a Hospital Setting in Bay Area where he works with patient who suffer from mental health problems.

He also has a small private practice where his focus is treatment of insomnia and mental health problem.

INTRODUCTION

Imagine you had a busy day at work. You came home and spent time with your family or significant other. You took care of your remaining work in the evening. When it's time to go to sleep, you worry that this will be another night where you will not be able to sleep well and fret over if you will have to wait for a long time to fall asleep. You are thinking about how you will feel the next day and how it can affect you and your work.

You get into bed, read a book, check your social media on your phone, and then try to sleep, but you can't go to sleep right away. You keep trying hard to go to sleep, but the effort is futile as you toss and turn. You keep thinking about why you can't sleep well. You finally go to sleep after being in bed for more than an hour, still having to wake up early in the morning to make sure you reach your office on time.

People who suffer from problems with insomnia (trouble going to sleep, waking up a lot, not feeling refreshed in the morning) go through the scenario mentioned above quite often. It is not easy to go through your night worrying about whether you can sleep and how long it will take you to fall asleep in the first place.

Problems with sleep affect our physical and mental health. It causes us to have issues in our social, family, and work lives.

In this book, we will give you the tools to help you sleep well. The program will focus on educating you about sleep problems. We will talk about different techniques to calm yourself down, so you don't feel too stressed out when you go to sleep. We will also talk about how to fill a Sleep Diary and the importance of a Sleep Diary. We will talk about the importance of Cognitive Behavioral Therapy, about Sleep Restriction, and Sleep Efficiency. We will also talk about Mindfulness.

This book will not only help you with your sleep but also help you have a better quality of life by teaching you the tools to help you focus on the present moment and to control your stress better.

CHAPTER 1

WHY INSOMNIA IS SO IMPORTANT

We spend almost 30% to 35% of our whole life sleeping. There is no human being who does not sleep during their life span. Without good sleep quality, we don't enjoy the quality of life we could have if we were to actually sleep well. Poor sleep causes many problems, not only physically and mentally, but it also affects our relationships, work, and family life.

We are so used to sleeping every night that we don't even think about sleep until we start having trouble with it. Once we have problems with our sleep, it is then that we realize what a blessing it is to have a peaceful night's rest.

Unfortunately, in this fast-paced world we spend very little time thinking about our sleep health. We try to sleep less during the week to catch up on our studies, or we work excessively to make sure we don't miss any deadlines at our jobs. We then try to catch up on our sleep on weekends. We put so much strain on our bodies up to the point that our bodies start showing signs of weakness, and we start developing medical and mental health problems.

Individuals who suffer from depression tend to have insomnia. If insomnia is not treated, even if their mood is treated, the chances of having them have a relapse of depression and depressive symptoms is high. If someone is sleeping better, it will help with their stress management, depression, and anxiety. There is also evidence that better sleep helps in managing chronic medical conditions as well.

More than 1/3 of the adult population has problems going to sleep, staying asleep, or waking up with poor quality of sleep.

Untreated insomnia can also cause increased anxiety, and people become at high risk for developing substance abuse disorders. People are also at high risk of developing depression if insomnia is left untreated.

If people are not getting a good quality of sleep, they have lower productivity at work and do not have a good quality of life. Their social and family life also gets affected by their lack of proper sleep. One research showed that insomnia is causing $63.2 billion a year in lost productivity.

Sleeping less than 5 hours per night can cause weight gain. Due to getting less sleep, we have a lower concentration of Leptin hormone (which signals the brain to let it know that you are full). When Leptin concentration is low, people eat more. Due to less sleep, we also have an increased concentration of the Ghrelin hormone (which stimulates appetite), so we tend to eat more when we are sleeping less.

People with insomnia are 28% more likely to develop Type 2 Diabetes. One research showed that compared to people who sleep 7-8 hours, people who sleep less have an increased risk of death of 12%. People are at risk of developing many medical problems due to untreated insomnia, and these include stroke, high blood pressure, obesity, and asthma.

CHAPTER 2

DEFINITION OF INSOMNIA

We all experience stressful life events such as moving, changing jobs, going through a divorce, medical problems, a family member not doing well, traveling, etc. These can cause us not to sleep well, but it's usually transient, and our sleep gets better as our mind and body heal, and we are able to sleep better. If sleep problems persist longer than three months, though, then we are developing insomnia, and we need to get help for it.

People who suffer from insomnia have difficulty falling asleep and/or they are waking up a lot throughout the night. When people wake up during the night, they then have a hard time going to sleep. Some people have an early morning awakening and are unable to go back to sleep.

Trouble with sleep is persistent even if the person has the adequate opportunity and circumstances to go to sleep.

With insomnia, trouble sleeping occurs at least three times a week and persist for at least three months.

Due to the individual not being able to have a good quality of sleep, they have difficulty functioning during the day, with symptoms like low energy, poor focus, problem doing tasks at work, headaches, and feeling tired.

Everyone has different sleep requirements. Most people need between 6-8 hours of sleep. The average person usually goes to bed between 10–11 pm and wakes up around 6–8 am.

CHAPTER 3

SLEEP PHASES

Let's quickly go through the phases of sleep so we can have a better understanding of in which phase we have our deep sleep, in which phase we have our dreams, and why if we don't sleep well for few nights, our body can catch up on sleep.

Stage I: This is the first stage where you are in between wakefulness and sleepiness. Your body is relaxing, and you have rolling eye movements. Your respiration and your heart rate are slowing. Like when you are watching a boring movie, and your eyes are closing, and your head is drifting down, this is the first stage of sleep.

Stage II: From Stage 1, you enter Stage 2, which is deeper than Stage 1. You spend around 30-45 minutes in this stage.

Stage III and IV: This is the deepest stage of sleep. It's difficult to wake up at this stage. This stage is very important for renewing our physical energy for the next day. This stage is also very important for our immune system.

REM Sleep: This is the stage in which we dream. Our heart rate and breathing rate elevate in this stage. Males have a penile erection in this stage as well. REM sleep is also very important for our memory. REM sleep duration usually remains stable throughout life, although it decreases slightly in older age.

On a typical night, we spent 90 minutes in each of these five stages. On average, we have 4-6 of these 90-minute cycles. During the initial period of sleep, deep sleep lasts longer (around 1 hour), and REM sleep duration is shorter. As the night progresses, REM duration increases, and deep sleep (stages 3 and 4) decreases.

CHAPTER 4

HOW MUCH SLEEP DO I ACTUALLY NEED?

The majority of the young and adult populations need between 7-9 hours of sleep.

This is true for around 90% of the population. However, there are a few percentages of the population that will need little less than 7 hours or a little more than 10 hours of sleep.

As we progress in our lives, we tend to need less sleep:

A newborn (0-3 months) will sleep around 14-17 hours per day.

Preschoolers (ages 3-5 years) will need 10-13 hours of sleep.

School-age children (ages 6-13 years) will need 9-11 hours of sleep.

Teenagers (ages 14-17 years) will need 8-10 hours of sleep.

Older adults (65 years and onwards) will need 7-8 hours of sleep each day.

CAUSES OF INSOMNIA

There are three main causes of insomnia:

HOMEOSTATIC DISRUPTION

For people who suffer from insomnia, their body is not usually tired at the end of the day, and that can make them unable to go to sleep. Let's think about our Homeostasis of the body as a bicycle tire, and we need it to be inflated to go to sleep. To make it inflated, we must keep our bodies physically active. If we spend too much time in bed, lying or resting a lot during the daytime, then the tire will not be properly inflated, and we will not be able to rest well.

Homeostatic disruption causes reduced deep sleep drive because the body is not tired enough. Spending too much time in bed, napping frequently, and not being physically active during the daytime can cause

Sleep Like a Winner! Treatment of Insomnia

that. Sleep Restriction will help with curing this disruption. (We will talk more about *Sleep Restriction* later in the book.)

People with insomnia have a tendency to wake up later on the weekends, or if they have a poor night's sleep, they wake up late or stay in bed longer. They have this false belief that if they didn't sleep well, then they will have a bad day, which is actually not right. Staying in bed longer or not waking up at a consistent time causes their body to create an artificial jetlag-like set of symptoms, and they have problems with focus, increased anxiety, and increased irritability the next day.

People during the weekend spend time in bed or on the couch to "rest," to "relax," to "catch up on their low energy," etc. Some people even spend up to 6-8 hours each day on weekends on the couch. Do they feel more energetic or less energetic after doing that? *Less* energetic. By staying on the couch, your body is not tired, and you will have even more trouble going to sleep at night.

CIRCADIAN RHYTHM TROUBLE

There are people whose bodies adjust well or quickly to different times of sleep or traveling to different time zones. People with insomnia need to make sure that they go to sleep and wake up at the same time. Their bodies can also take a longer time to adjust if they travel to a different time zone.

In this busy world, we tend to sleep less to catch up on our work and try to "catch up" on our sleep during the weekends. We tend to sleep longer hours during weekends and sometimes go to bed later and wake up later. People with insomnia can have Circadian rhythm problems due to sleeping and waking up at different times during the week and weekends.

INCREASED AROUSAL

People with insomnia worry about going to sleep. They feel that once they go to bed, they will have trouble sleeping, and this might wake them up even more. The feeling of not being able to sleep causes people to get more anxious and, in turn, causes more insomnia. They try very hard to go to sleep, but most of the time, they are unsuccessful. The harder they try, the harder it becomes for them to fall asleep; they get more frustrated, and that causes a vicious cycle where the harder they try, the worse their sleep problem gets.

Doing physically strenuous activity or exercising too close to bedtime can also cause the body to be active and, in turn, cause problems with sleep.

Stimulus Control, *Sleep Hygiene*, *Relaxation*, and *Cognitive Therapy* will help with Increased Arousal. (We will talk more about these later in the book.)

CHAPTER 6

TOOLS TO DIAGNOSE INSOMNIA

There are few different ways to diagnose insomnia. The most common one that we usually hear is to conduct a "sleep study". Sleep studies don't usually pick-up insomnia very well, as most people with insomnia have a hard time going to sleep or staying asleep in the sleep lab. Sleep studies are more effective at diagnosing other sleep disorders such as sleep apnea, but not insomnia.

These days, people wear smartwatches and Fitbit trackers that have many uses. They monitor people's activity levels, and that helps people to gauge how many calories they have burned during their daily activities. Smartwatches and Fitbit trackers are great for monitoring your daytime activity, but, unfortunately, they are not very good at monitoring your sleep.

These devices calculate sleep by monitoring a person's activity levels. People go to bed while wearing these devices and lay down. The devices think that the person is sleeping as there is no physical activity, even though the person is only laying down in bed and waiting to sleep without having drifted off yet. People with insomnia stay in bed for a long time (not a good idea) until they can fall asleep, and the device overestimates the sleep time. The same thing happens when they are awake but laying in bed, not moving. Again, the device thinks that the person is sleeping, and then it underestimates the time the person is awake.

The best tool to diagnose insomnia is a Sleep Diary/Sleep Log. It is an excellent tool to track how many hours you slept, how long it took you to go to sleep, how much time it took you to get out of bed, etc. Ideally, 14 days of sleep tracking will be helpful so it can show a better data point. A person should not worry about filling their sleep diary out at night, as it can cause some anxiety, so the best time is to focus on filling it in after you wake up in the morning. Try not to overthink about it and fill it quickly.

CHAPTER 7

CONDITIONS THAT ARE "NOT INSOMNIA"

OBSTRUCTIVE SLEEP APNEA (OSA)

People with insomnia are "tired," but usually, they are not "sleepy." They have restlessness that can make them upset easily due to not able to sleep well, but people with Obstructive Sleep Apnea (OSA) have "excessive daytime sleepiness."

The Epworth Sleepiness Scale is a good scale to rule out whether you have excessive daytime sleepiness. You can find the scale easily by searching with Google or Yahoo. A score that is greater than 10 means that you are more likely to have excessive daytime sleepiness compared to just restlessness or exhaustion.

People with OSA have excessive daytime sleepiness. During their impaired sleep, they have trouble breathing. Their trouble breathing generally lasts for about 10 seconds, and this usually causes them to wake up. This can occur a minimum of five times each hour.

In moderate to extreme cases, people can wake up frequently (even every few minutes) due to the blockage of air. The reason they wake up is due to the brain not being able to get oxygen, so they wake up to breathe air.

People with OSA can also have chronic insomnia, but a person needs to get OSA treatment first before they get insomnia treatment. OSA is a potentially life-threatening condition and can cause death.

People can have multiple comorbid issues related to OSA, such as depression, headache, heart problems, high blood pressure, weight gain, and muscle aches.

OSA Risk Factors:

- Excessive tiredness or sleepiness during daytime (Epworth score >10)

- Observed to have stopped breathing at night and snores heavily

- Elevated blood pressure

- BMI greater than 35

- Age greater than 50

- Neck circumference of greater than 17cm in males and greater than 16cm in females

- The male gender has a higher rate of occurrence (2:1 ratio of male to female cases)

CIRCADIAN RHYTHM SLEEP DISORDERS

Delayed sleep phase

People with delayed sleep phase have a hard time going to sleep and usually are only able to go to sleep 3-4 hours later than the average population, typically going to bed around 12–1 am and waking up around 7–8 am.

Advanced sleep phase

People with advanced sleep phase have a hard time keeping themselves awake, and they tend to go to sleep around 8–9 pm and wake up around 4–5 am. They usually complain about waking up too early.

RESTLESS LEG SYNDROME

People who suffer from Restless Leg Syndrome feel that when they go to sleep, they have the uncontrollable urge to move their feet; due to this, they have problems with their sleep. It can also happen even when they are sitting. Most of the time, it happens in the evening or nighttime. They need to get outside the bed and move their feet to get some relief.

This condition can be caused by low iron, pregnancy, a complication of diabetes, or some other neurological problem. Depending on the cause, the treatment varies from medication treatment to managing the underlying disorder causing Restless Leg Syndrome (RLS).

CHAPTER 8

INSOMNIA RATING SCALE

Let's rate our insomnia severity to find out just how bad our insomnia is. This will help us to have a benchmark as well, so we can continue to come back to that scale during treatment to find out if the severity of our insomnia is getting better. Ideally, we would like this severity rating to be less over time, decreasing as we progress through the program.

Insomnia Rating Scale

Please rate it on a scale of 1-10, where 1 is no problem and 10 is very severe

	Before program	After finishing the program
Problem going to sleep		
Problem staying asleep		
Waking up too early		
Worrying about if I can sleep		
Affecting my Relationship		
Affecting my work		
Affecting my social life		
Total		

When you finish the program, come back and use the Insomnia Rating Scale again to see if the scale indicates a lower score. I am very hopeful that if you follow the book, you will see significant improvement in your scores.

CHAPTER 9

SLEEP LOGS

Keeping logs of your sleep is one of the most accurate ways to monitor how you are sleeping, how often you are waking up, how much time it is taking you to fall asleep, how long you stay in bed, and your total time of sleep.

Ideally, we would like to get two weeks' worth of data to figure which aspect of insomnia you'll need to work on most. For example, if you are spending too much time in bed after you wake up, that can cause problems with sleep the next day. If you are going to bed and unable to sleep but are "trying" hard to go to sleep, then you need to work on not spending too much time "trying" to go to sleep.

Remember that you are estimating the times, so you don't have to obsessively check the clock. Make sure that you don't have access to the clock in the room, but if you have access, try not to look at it. You can focus on jotting down things in your sleep diary when you wake up in the morning.

You will need at least one week of data (but ideally two weeks' worth).

Sample Sleep Log:

	Mon	Tue	Wed	Thu	Fri	Sat	Sun
Went to Bed	0900 pm	0930 pm	0900 pm	0930 pm	1000 pm	1100pm	0930 pm
Fell Asleep	0930 pm	1000 pm	1000 pm	1000 pm	1100 pm	1130 pm	1000 pm
How many times awake during night	2	1	1	1	1	1	1
Total time awake during night	60 min	30 min	60 min	30 min	30 min	30 min	30 min
Wake up time	6:00 am	6:30 am	6:00 am	6:30 am	6:30 am	8:30 am	9:30 am
Came out from bed	0630 am	0700 am	0700 am	0700 am	0700 am	0900 am	0930 am
Total time spend in bed	9:30 hrs	9:30 hrs	10:00 hrs	9:30 hrs	9:00 hrs	10:00 hrs	12:00 hrs
Total sleep time	7:30 hrs	8:00 hrs	7:00 hrs	8:00 hrs	7:00 hrs	8:30 hrs	11:00 hrs

As I mentioned before, you don't have to be completely accurate in regard to timing. Just make reasonable time estimates, and once you do so for 1-2 weeks, we will have fairly good data to work with.

When jotting information in the sleep log, remember that you will start "Went to sleep" on Monday night and will write the "Came out from bed" time in the Monday section as well, even though you technically woke up on Tuesday morning.

You can calculate the total amount of time you spent in bed by adding the hours you spent in bed from the moment you "went to bed" (Monday at 9 pm) to the time you "came out from bed" (Tuesday 6:30 am). So, in total, you spent 9:30 hours.

You can calculate total sleep time by first finding your total time in bed (Monday 9:30 hours) and then sub-tracting it from the time it took you to go to sleep (Monday 30 minutes), total time awake during the night (Monday 60 min/1hour), and time spent to get out from bed (Monday 30 minutes) which is: (9:30 hours) − (30 min + 60 min + 30 min) = 7:30 hours.

Let's quickly talk about Sleep Efficiency while we are talking about the Sleep Log: it refers to the percentage of the time that a person is asleep. This percentage is calculated by dividing the total sleep time by the total time in bed. Let's calculate Sleep Efficiency from above the Sleep Log.

On Monday, your total sleep time was 7:30 hours (450 minutes).

The total time in bed was 9:30 hours (570 minutes).

Sleep Efficiency was: (450/570) multiply 100 = 78.94%.

Now you can start logging your sleep in the Sleep Log.

You don't have to start on Monday; you can start any day. Once you have 1-2 weeks of data, you can start working on the sleep techniques that we will discuss later on in the book.

	Mon	Tue	Wed	Thu	Fri	Sat	Sun
Went to Bed							
Fell Asleep							
How many times awake during night							
Total time awake during night							
Wake up time							
Came out from bed							
Total time spend in bed							
Total sleep time							

CHAPTER 10

DAILY MONITORING

While you are noticing your sleep patterns in the daily logs and throughout the remaining course of the sleep training, I would like you to do "Daily Monitoring," ideally in the evening but not too close to your bedtime. This daily monitoring, like the Sleep Log, will help you tremendously in keeping track of your physical activity, diet, caffeine consumption, smoking habits, and mood tracking. It will also provide linear data to show if your Daily Habits are getting better as you progress through the program. You will also work on your Daily Habits that can hinder your sleep.

Here is the Daily Monitoring Log:

DAILY MONITORING	Sample	Mon	Tue	Wed	Thur	Fri	Sat	Sun
Exercise								
Total caffeine used								
Last consumption of caffeinated product								
Alcohol use								
Smoking								
Last meal of the day								
Tiredness level (1-10 level 3 times a day)								
Mood (1-10 level)								

CHAPTER 11

SLEEP HYGIENE

In this chapter, we will talk about sleep hygiene, as it not only helps us sleep better but also helps with a better quality of life. We know most of the stuff we will talk about in this chapter, but sometimes we need constant reminders to make sure we do certain things. Sometimes we need to re-read material, so we continue to follow these habits in our life.

Exercising will not only help with your sleep but will also help with your physical and mental health. Sometimes, especially during the weekends, we spend a lot of time on media or the computer, or we binge on TV, and that can cause us to not be physically active.

When we are not physically active, our bodies are not physically and mentally tired, and that can cause us not to sleep well during the night.

There is no perfect time to exercise, but I recommend for people to exercise in the morning. The advantage of exercising in the morning is that you have fewer distractions, your body is not tired, exercising helps to activate your body in the mornings, you will have better concentration to tackle your mornings at work, and you don't have to worry about exercise later in the day if you are coming home late from work and feeling tired.

Some people feel that they like to exercise after work as they feel more relaxed that they don't have to worry about going to work, and they have more energy in the evenings. In general, people vary, so there is no perfect answer regarding when to exercise. The goal should just be that you do it consistently.

Make sure not to exercise close to bedtime as it can stimulate your brain and can cause problems with your sleep. If you feel that you are exercising late in the day and that you are having trouble with sleep, consider changing your exercise time schedule.

Make sure that throughout the day, you are taking frequent breaks at work and stretching your body. Take short walks during your work breaks. During lunch, go outside, even If it's only for five minutes. Every 30 minutes stand up and walk for 2-3 minutes or stretch a little.

I like to have at least one cup of tea in the morning and a cup of coffee in the afternoon. People who suffer from insomnia can drink caffeine, but they need to be mindful of how much they drink, making sure not to drink caffeinated products too late in the day.

If you drink caffeine, don't consume more than 300 mg of caffeine per day (equivalent to three 8oz cups of coffee). Avoid coffee in the latter part of the evening as coffee Is a stimulant. It is also an adenosine blocker, so it can also lead to less depth in your sleep. You also don't want to drink any caffeine after 2 pm if your sleep time is 9 pm. (Ideally, avoid caffeine 6-7 hours from your bedtime.)

Drinking alcohol can help you go to sleep and relax your body, but you will be waking up more during the night, and the deep sleep phase of your sleep will be reduced. You may not feel refreshed upon waking up the next day.

People who drink alcohol on a daily basis can also have alcohol withdrawal symptoms in their sleep, and that can cause even more disturbance. Does that mean you shouldn't drink? You can consume alcohol but try not to drink excessively and daily. Also, try not to drink too close to your bedtime.

Avoid eating heavy meals close to your bedtime as well. Try to use mindful eating habits as it will help you eat more healthily and avoid overeating. When you eat, look closely at what you are eating: look at the texture of the food, smell the food, enjoy the taste of each bite, and chew well. Eat slowly and enjoy every bite. If you feel hungry at bedtime, drink some milk or have some oatmeal or fruit.

CHAPTER 12

SLEEP-INDUCING ENVIRONMENT

In an ideal world, you would like to use your bed only for sleep and for intimacy. If you have insomnia, then you definitely need to make sure that you don't use your bed aside for sleep and intimacy. If you like to read before you go to sleep, be sure it is not causing you to have problems with sleep, and make sure not to read for an extended period of time in your bed before going to sleep.

Avoid using cell phones, watching TV, or browsing the internet at least an hour before you go to sleep. If you have to use electronic devices, then consider using them in a low or dim light setting.

Clean your room to make it feel cozy and remove clutter. You want to create a room where, whenever you enter, you feel relaxed and feel like sleeping.

If you like particular scents or calming music to help you with your sleep, then consider using them. Aromatherapy can relax your brain and calm you down so you can sleep better.

If you are working indoors or don't have access to natural sunlight, consider using a lightbox early in the morning for 20-30 minutes each day. You can find lightboxes on Amazon or from medical supply stores in your area.

Drink plenty of water during the day but avoid drinking too much at night; otherwise, you will wake up in the middle of the night needing to use the restroom.

Keep your room quiet and cool. Set a comfortable temperature in your room; the ideal temperature is in the mid-60s (Fahrenheit).

Make sure you have a comfortable mattress and pillow. If you find that you wake up with neck or back stiffness, consider changing your pillow or mattress to something that offers better support.

Take a warm shower before you go to bed. Some people feel rejuvenated and alert after a warm shower, so if you are the type to do so, don't try taking a shower before you go to bed unless you feel it will relax you.

There is also research showing that certain bedroom colors like blue, green, and yellow can help with sleep.

CHAPTER 13

SLEEP LOSS

People with insomnia feel "tired," but most of the time, they are not sleepy. They can function reasonably well, although doing things will take more effort and require more motivation to do so. They might also feel "upset" or "irritable" due to not sleeping well. They also sometimes feel that they have not "done enough" or "not done as well" as they would have done if they had slept well.

Even If people don't sleep well for few days, they usually recover most of the deep sleep (stage 3 and stage 4). Remember from our earlier discussion that this is the stage that is very important for renewing our physical energy, and it also helps with our immune systems.

In this program, we will talk about the different techniques that will help you with your sleep. Remember that attempting to force yourself to sleep does not work. It's like running after your own shadow. The more you run after it, the more it will run from you.

CHAPTER 14

SLEEP REGULATORY SYSTEM

There are two systems in our body that work together to help us sleep well. If we have an imbalance in one of the systems, then we will not be able to sleep properly.

HOMEOSTATIC SYSTEM: This system compensates for lost sleep by increasing the amount of deep sleep that a person usually gets. Usually, the more active you are during the daytime, the deeper sleep you will get in the homeostatic system. If a person who has trouble sleeping tries to sleep earlier in the day, then he/she is not as active during the daytime and will have decreased rejuvenation from the homeostatic system.

CIRCADIAN RHYTHM: We usually call it our "body clock," and it is the one that tells the body when it's time to go to bed and when It's time to wake up. Light exposure at nighttime can disrupt this system and cause us to be more awake; therefore, it's better to avoid screen time before going to sleep.

The average person usually takes between 10-30 minutes to go to sleep and ideal Sleep efficiency is around 85% and above.

CHAPTER 15

TRUST THE TREATMENT!

There is significant research that shows the effectiveness of Cognitive Behavioral Therapy (CBT) for insomnia. The treatment will take time, but you will eventually be able to sleep well. Most people start noticing improvement within 2-3 weeks, so the first few weeks will be a bit difficult.

You need to trust the process in order to make it work. If you feel that the treatment will not work and you keep telling yourself that you have tried many different treatments in the past without success, then it might not be successful as you are conditioning your brain against the process.

During the difficult times while you are doing this course, remember that rough patches will come, but if you persist, then you will feel better. There may be days where you will feel upset or sad. There may be days that you will take naps during the daytime. There may be days that you will not enjoy the social gatherings that you used to enjoy but hang in there, my friend. Things will get better.

CHAPTER 16

PREPARING TO START TREATMENT

Our body has a mechanism to take care of lost sleep. When you lose sleep, the next night, the body spends more time in deep sleep and in the dream sleep phase that can help our body to feel energetic the next day.

We think that if we lie down in bed even if we cannot sleep, then "relaxing" in bed will help us to go to sleep. The fact is that the harder you try to go to sleep, the more difficult it will be to actually do so. If you cannot sleep, come out of bed rather than still lying down as it will not only cause further trouble with sleep, but it will also make you more frustrated.

You will need about 2-3 weeks to start feeling better if you follow the sleep treatment.

1-2 weeks prior to starting the treatment, you are focusing on gathering data regarding your sleep.

Make sure that you start the program when you are not traveling, you don't have any extra stress occurring, and your work life is not too busy.

You don't have to start the program on a Monday. Some people like to start the program on a Thursday or Friday.

You don't have to take time off to do this program either. It's better that you have a specific plan to keep yourself busy (e.g., cooking, walking, meeting with people, reading, watching movies, etc.) before you start the program as sometimes people have a hard time during the afternoons, especially when they are at home. Most of the time, increased sedation happens between 1–4 pm during the day.

Discuss your plans with your family members so they are aware that, for the next few weeks, you may be leaving the room when you cannot sleep.

You can also talk to people at work about the fact that you are starting a sleep program. Informing them that if you appear tired for the next few days, then it's due to the fact that you are adjusting your sleep cycle.

If you feel that you are feeling "sleepy" and are nodding off, then it is best to avoid operating any heavy machinery or driving a car.

Naps are prohibited during the course of the treatment, but if you absolutely have to take a nap, don't take it for more than 30 minutes. If you are taking naps, consider taking them before 3:00 or 3:30 pm.

This treatment does not work if someone is having unstable moods, such as manic/hypomanic episodes in bipolar disorder or a psychotic episode. In this program you will also need to restrict your sleep, and that can cause an exacerbation of mood problems.

Medical problems like seizure disorder can be triggered, especially when you are restricting your sleep, so it's better if you have a condition like this to consult with your doctor before considering sleep restriction.

CHAPTER 17

TREATMENT MINDSET

Treatment of insomnia not only helps people with improving their sleep quality, but it also helps them to have a better quality of life. It gives them more control in their life, and they are more productive. You will also be able to manage your day-to-day stressors better by learning cognitive behavioral therapy tools.

You will be able to live in the moment, and hopefully, your mind will not be thinking about things that you don't have any control over. You learn to radically accept the things over which you have control and the things you do not. When you feel better and more in control of your life, you also begin to feel that the world around you looks better, and your frustration tolerance will improve. People around you will also feel happier as they will feel more positive energy from you. Remember that the treatment of insomnia is within you, and you need persistence and resilience for the treatment to work.

For any training to work, you first need to have trust in the training and be willing to do the work. For example, you can hire a personal trainer, but if you don't have trust in the trainer and are not willing to put in the work, you will not be able to see any change in your physical health.

For this sleep training to work, you first have to believe that sleep medications are an easy temporary fix for few days, but they will not solve the overall problem. You will feel better after 4-6 weeks of sleep training, and then you will be sleeping well for the rest of your life. Imagine sleeping well for the rest of your entire life but only needing to put in the effort for 4-6 weeks to make it happen!

CHAPTER 18

TREATING INSOMNIA

As we know, the non-pharmaceutical approach is the best approach to treat insomnia. You can use it whenever you like it, and it does not need a "prescription" from any provider. It does not have any side effects except during the first few days when you will feel tired and may experience difficulty with focusing. You don't have to worry about dependence on any medications nor worry about handling withdrawal symptoms if you were to ever run out of those medications.

If you are taking sleep aids, that does not mean you cannot take advantage of this treatment as well. People using sleep aids can reduce or completely stop sleep medications after finishing this treatment program. I do recommend consulting with your medical provider before you consider tapering down or stopping any of your medications, though, as you will need to be monitored closely by your provider.

There are four ways to tackle insomnia, and you will need to apply all four of those concepts/applications to your daily sleep regimen to get the maximum results from the program.

These four concepts are: Stimulus Control, Sleep Restriction, Cognitive Restructuring, and Relaxation Techniques.

STIMULUS CONTROL (B OF CBTI):

Stimulus control is part of the behavioral component of Cognitive Behavioral Therapy for Insomnia (CBTi). The main reason to do it is to train your brain to associate the bed with sleep only. It takes time to train your brain to do that, and usually, a person needs to do it at least 2-3 weeks before they can start seeing the benefits from it. It's not easy, but it does work!

In stimulus control, you have to make sure you only use the bed for sleep or for intimacy. You should not lie down once you are awake. As soon as you are awake, you should come out of bed. You want to train your brain that whenever you see your bed, It should only think about either sleep or intimacy - nothing else.

You should go to bed and get out of bed at the same time each day, even if you don't feel that you've gotten enough sleep. Even on weekends, you will follow the same regimen.

You will only go to bed when you are about to fall asleep. If you cannot fall asleep, you need to get up from the bed. You will not be taking any daytime naps.

You will also not read, watch TV, or use the computer in your bed. You will have to decrease the brightness on your TV and computer screen if you do have to use the screen at night but consider not using it at all at least an hour before you go to bed.

Don't try to watch shows that can stimulate you too much, like an action movie, or do intense things like finishing up a work project that will require a lot of brain activity. If you do need to take care of some things or indulge in a hobby, you can try to find a place in your house where you can sit, relax, and read. Once you are tired, you can stand up and walk to your bed to sleep.

If you cannot fall asleep, you need to get up and lie/sit on that comfortable chair/sofa.

Remember, it will not be easy to go to bed and wake up at the same time each day. You may feel tired the next day, but you have to make sure to avoid taking any naps. If you do absolutely have to take a nap, try taking it for no longer than 30 minutes, and try to do so before 3:30 pm.

You may have a hard time getting out of your bed when you wake up, and you may think that you should lie down for just 10–15 more minutes, but you have to train your brain, and you have to give the brain the same signal every day, so you need to get up.

You can even get up and go lie down on your couch for few minutes if you need to. Or you could stand up, drink a glass of water, do some stretches, or get out of your bed and say to yourself, "I had adequate sleep last night," or "Let's face this amazing day!"

SLEEP RESTRICTION THERAPIES (B OF CBTI):

To increase your sleep drive, we use Sleep Restriction Therapy (SRT). This is also a behavioral component of CBTi. In simple words, it's the amount of time you spend in bed. You would like to have a good quality of sleep rather than a long quantity of time in bed. You would rather sleep six hours straight than be in bed for hours and get six hours of frequent-wakefulness sleep. If you are able to achieve deep sleep, you will feel refreshed.

To do that, you need to review your 2-week sleep diary and calculate the total sleep time and the total time in bed. Average both together, and you will come up with a number.

For example, you have your average total sleep time of 6:30 hours and total time in bed of 8:30 hours. You then have to figure out what time you would like to wake up, and then you will add 30 minutes to the total sleep time.

Two weeks of Sleep Data:

	Average
Went to Bed	11pm
Fell Asleep	11:30pm
How many times awake during night	2
Total time awake during night	60 min
Wake up time	7:00am
Came out from bed	7:30am
Total time spend in bed	08:30
Total sleep time	06:30

In the earlier sections we talked about how to calculate your total sleep time. Lets do it again:

You can calculate total sleep time by first finding your total time in bed (8:30 hours)

and

then subtracting it from the time it took you to go to sleep (30 minutes), total time awake during the night (60 min/1hour), and time spent to get out from bed (30 minutes) which is 120 minutes or 2 hours.

So the total sleep time is:

(8:30 hours) – (30 min + 60 min + 30 min) = 6:30 hours

In this example your total sleep time is 6:30 hours.

You will add 30 minutes to the total sleep time, so it's now 7 hours.

Now, you will go to bed at 12 am to wake up at 7 am.

Let's look at another person's 2-week Sleep Diary to clarify if you have any confusion about the Sleep Logs.

	Average
Went to Bed	9:00pm
Fell Asleep	10:00pm
How many times awake during night	1
Total time awake during night	60 min
Wake up time	7:00am
Came out from bed	8:00am
Total time spend in bed	11hours
Total sleep time	8hours

Average total sleep time last week: 8 hours. We will add 30 minutes to this to make it 0830 hours. Reason for adding 30 minutes is because it usually takes around 10-15 minutes to go to sleep so that's why for now, we are keeping 30 minutes extra time to make sure a person is getting adequate amount of sleep.

New sleep time: 10:30 pm (8:30 hours total sleep if you sleep at 10:30 pm and wake up at 0700 am).

The reason we are keeping wake up time the same is because you have control over when you wake up, and you can set an alarm for that. Initially, it's difficult to know when you will be able to sleep since your body will take some time to adjust to going to sleep.

Remember: it will be difficult to adjust to this time frame at first, and lots of people feel "tired" and "sleepy," but hang in there and keep yourself occupied. You can ask your friend, children, or partner to be with you and talk to you, so you don't fall asleep before the allocated time to go to bed.

Usually, it's better to have less usage of cellphones/ tablets, but if you have trouble keeping yourself awake, then you should use electronics for a little while to make sure you have some stimulating activity to keep yourself awake.

Gradually, the sleep time will be increased by 15-30 minutes if you feel very sleepy during the daytime but are also sleeping well during the nighttime without spending too much time in bed to go to sleep (sleeping within 10-15 minutes of going to bed) and following a strict sleep regimen like waking up and going to bed at the same time.

CHAPTER 19

WEEK 1 (WORRY TIME, MINDFULNESS BASICS)

Congratulations! You are on your first week!

You have compiled your 1-2 week of Sleep Log Data and have calculated how many hours you will be sleeping. You have also decided that you will not spend time in bed except for sleep or being intimate with your partner. You will make sure that you keep yourself away from screen time at least an hour before you go to bed. If you do have to use a cellphone, watch TV, or work on the computer, be sure to have it set to less light/brightness.

Make sure to fill this week's Sleep Log. As we discussed earlier, you don't have to be perfect and just have to roughly guess at what times you slept and woke up. Make sure that you don't look at the clock at nighttime, as this can cause even more anxiety. Have the room dim at night. Let your family/significant other know that you are starting your sleep treatment as of this week.

	Mon	Tue	Wed	Thu	Fri	Sat	Sun
Went to Bed							
Fell Asleep							
How many times awake during night							
Total time awake during night							
Wake up time							
Came out from bed							
Total time spend in bed							
Total sleep time							
Sleep Efficiency							

People will also need some motivation to wake up in the morning, such as Behavioral Activation that focuses on Exercise/Meditation in the morning. A lot of times, when we wake up, our energy levels are down, and we "wait for energy" to be there before getting out of bed. The problem with that thinking is that you need to be active to have more energy, as movement creates energy and "action will cause you to feel more motivated."

Some other activities that can stimulate you are walking outside, opening the room's blinds, taking a shower, drinking warm tea, drinking water, and drinking warm tea with honey.

I have personally used light box therapy when I lived in states where it was very cold and snowed a lot. I noticed my energy levels were very low in the morning, and my mood was down. Sitting in front of a lightbox for 20-30 minutes makes a big difference in energy levels and mood. You can make your breakfast and eat it with your lightbox in front of you. These days you can get very reasonably priced lightboxes from online stores like Amazon.

Remember, positive things will only happen when you come out of your comfort zone, and in the case right now, the comfort zone is your bed.

This is your first week so try to have a lesser load at your work if possible. You would like to have less stress at work so you can focus on your sleep for the next couple of weeks. I also recommend not to take on any new projects for the next couple of weeks.

Try to be social with friends but not spend too much time outside the home as you need to go to bed at the same time each day.

During the weekends, be sure that you keep yourself busy. Ideally, you should plan your weekend ahead with pleasurable activities, so you have less time to worry about things, as well as worry about your sleep.

Try to spend time outside the house doing things like walking, cycling, or going to the mall. If you are at home, consider not sitting in one spot for a long period of time. If you are watching TV or using the computer, try to stretch every 30-45 minutes or walk even for just a few minutes inside the house to keep your blood flowing and keep you alert.

If you are taking sleep medications on a regular basis, I recommend not stopping them during this phase of the treatment. Once you start sleeping better, consider cutting the dosage down gradually under the supervision of your doctor. Remember that if you taper down your medications and you have problems with insomnia, it does not mean the insomnia is back. Sometimes after stopping sleep medications, people can have rebound insomnia that can last for a few days to a few weeks, but it does get better.

IMPORTANT POINTS:

- Go to bed only when you are tired.
- Wake up at the same time even if you are tired.
- If you cannot sleep after 10-15 minutes in bed, then get up.
- Try not to take daytime naps.

From this week on, you will also start working on things you can do to help your hyperarousal state. There are many techniques to work with when it comes to the hyperarousal state. This week, you will work on a couple of those. The first one will be to schedule worry time, and the second one will be the introduction of mindfulness.

WORRY TIME:

We all worry; some people worry more and some less. The problem with excessive worry is that it feels like your mind keeps thinking about an issue without focusing on the current moment, and you are unable to spend any quality time.

If we worry about few things throughout the day, then the chances are that it will affect our mood and our quality of sleep. If you can fix the problem that is causing you to feel anxious, then fix it on the spot, but if you cannot fix the thing that is causing you to be worried, write it down on a piece of paper or put a note about it on your smartphone. Schedule a specific time of the day that you will intentionally worry about, and if you get any worry during the daytime, then tell yourself that you will worry during your scheduled "worry time."

In your worry time, you can worry, but also try to think about what other solutions to your problems may be or what some alternate thoughts that can help with the worry may be as well. It's better not to allot the worry time too late in the day as you might think too much around nighttime about the issues. Don't spend more than 15-20 minutes with your worry time. Try not to schedule it later at night as it can cause problems with your sleep. When you first put the worry time into your schedule, try to do so at 6 pm for 20 minutes, for example. You can set your alarm for 20 minutes. Make sure to also have a comfortable location inside or outside your home.

Review the Worry Log and think about possible solutions. It might be possible that some of the things in the worry log will not be a concern anymore, and you don't even have to work on it. If you cannot fix a problem right away, though, then move that worry to the next day.

MINDFULNESS:

We all are busy in our life, and most of the time, we are on autopilot mode. We wake up, do our hygiene rituals, eat breakfast, and drive to work. Our mind is constantly wandering to different thoughts throughout the day without focusing on the current moment. We think about the past and worry about the future, and we forget to live in the moment. If we think back on the major events in life like teaching our kids how to ride a bicycle, when we went to a baseball game, our wedding day, etc., we realize that the reason we remember most aspects of those events is because we were present mindfully during those events.

Most of the time, when our brain is wandering around, it's thinking about things that cause us to worry. That is why we need to bring our wandering mind back to the present moment, not only to live in the current moment but also to help us feel less anxious.

Living in the current moment does not mean that we will have pleasant sensations and feelings all the time. We will have moments that we will not like, but we need to accept how things are without judgment.

Consider doing 3-5 minutes of breathing exercises 1-3 times a day if you are new to this practice. When you do the breathing exercise, your mind will wander, but you need to gently bring it back to the current moment. This exercise is one of the basics but is still a very powerful exercise that will help you to be mindful and to be present in the moment.

You can do this breathing exercise by sitting on the floor or sitting on a chair. If you choose to sit on the floor, consider using a cushion. You can cross your legs comfortably at the ankle and don't necessarily have to place your feet on the opposite thighs. If you have chosen to sit on a chair, then be sure not to use the back of the chair for support.

Make sure to have good posture. You can keep your eyes closed as it can eliminate any external distraction. If you don't want to close your eyes, you can keep them open and find a spot around 5-6 feet away from your body that you can look at, so you don't get distracted.

Now you can simply start breathing in and breathing out. There are many ways that you can observe your breath. I usually observe that when I breathe in, my breath is cold, and when I breathe out, my breath is a little hot. Sometimes I also observe my abdomen expanding and contracting with each breath.

Try to focus on your breath. If you are new to this, you will see that your mind wanders a lot, but gently bring your mind back to the current moment and continue to focus on your breathing.

If you are short of time or have a hard time with this exercise, consider doing it only for 3-5 minutes in the beginning, even just once a day. As you get better with it and enjoy it more, you can increase the duration and frequency.

For the rest of the duration of the program, you will continue to do Worry Time and Breathing Exercises every day to get the maximum out of the course.

CHAPTER 20

WEEK 2 (SLEEP EFFICIENCY, COGNITIVE MODEL)

Congratulations on finishing your first week of Sleep Training. The first couple of weeks are the toughest ones, and things will start getting better after that. You should give yourself a treat for finishing your first week.

You also need to review how your first week went. Were you feeling excessively tired during the daytime and having increased urges to go to sleep? Were you able to go to sleep right away? Were you waking up a lot? Were you able to follow the sleep routine regularly?

If you didn't follow the sleep routine regularly, such as going to sleep at a different time than what you had decided, or you woke up later than the time you had decided, then I recommend now moving forward to week 2 and re-doing week 1. It's very common that, during the first week, people don't follow the treatment completely.

In week 2, we will first review our Sleep Diary from week one and then adjust our sleep time and duration. We will also discuss what Sleep Efficiency is. If you followed the sleep regimen completely, then look at the average of all your weekly times and plot it in this Sleep Log:

	Average
Went to Bed	
Fell Asleep	
How many times awake during night	
Total time awake during night	
Wake up time	
Came out from bed	
Total time spend in bed	
Total sleep time	
Sleep Efficiency	

HOW TO CALCULATE SLEEP EFFICIENCY:

Sleep Efficiency tells us the quality of sleep we are getting when we sleep at night. To calculate Sleep Efficiency, we will need to divide the total sleep time by the total time we spent in the bed and multiply it by 100 to get a percentage.

For example, if your total sleep time is 8 hours and your total time in bed is 10, your Sleep Efficiency is: (8/10) * 100 = 80%

Calculate Sleep Efficiency Formula: (total sleep time/ total time in bed) x 100

Once you have calculated your first week's Sleep Efficiency, then you can look at the following Sleep Efficiency chart to find out if you need to add, subtract, or continue at the same times as last week.

Sleep Efficiency	How much to change my sleep time
84% or less	Go to bed 15 minutes later
85% - 89%	Go to bed at the same time as last week
90%-94%	Go to bed 15 minutes earlier
95% or higher	Go to bed 30 minutes earlier

This week, you can again log your sleep time in the following Sleep Log:

	Mon	Tue	Wed	Thu	Fri	Sat	Sun
Went to Bed							
Fell Asleep							
How many times awake during night							
Total time awake during night							
Wake up time							
Came out from bed							
Total time spend in bed							
Total sleep time							
Sleep Efficiency							

This week we will also discuss a very important topic that will not only help you with your sleep but will also help you in many areas of your life: The Cognitive Model of Cognitive Behavioral Therapy.

According to Cognitive Behavioral Therapy (CBT), it's not the actual event that causes us to feel depressed; it's how we perceive those events or the meaning we give to those events.

The cognitive triangle is a triangle of thinking, feeling, and behavior. These three are interconnected to each other.

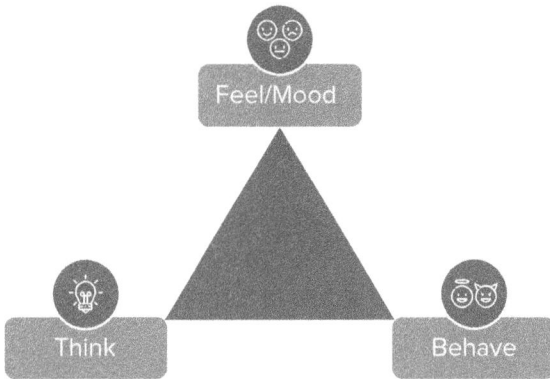

Our thinking, feeling, and behavior are interconnected. Each of these influence each other.

If you have thoughts like "I will not be able to sleep well," you will likely feel down and anxious, and that will make your body tense, and you will feel anxious when you go to bed. Once you are in bed, you may keep thinking, "I will not be able to sleep well," and in turn, this will make you toss and turn throughout the night.

If you are feeling good or optimistic, you may be thinking that "things will get better even I don't sleep well for a couple of nights," and that may make your body more relaxed. In turn, this can help you sleep better as now you are not worried if you sleep well or not because your brain is thinking that you will be fine even if you don't sleep well for a couple of nights, so there is no "pressure" to get a good night's sleep.

If you are in the behavioral part of the triangle, doing pleasurable activity will make you feel better, and that will help you not to think too much or to think more positively about stressors in your life.

Automatic Thoughts

Spontaneous
Usually brief and people don't notice them

Situation → Automatic Thoughts →

| Emotion |
| Behavior |
| Physiological |

Automatic thoughts are our thoughts that keep popping up all the time. They are usually brief, spontaneous, and most of the time, we don't notice them.

Imagine you are in a grocery store and the person in one of the aisles is moving very slowly; your automatic thought may be, "Doesn't he know that I am behind him? He should move fast!" or "He is making me reach home late!" or "People should buy stuff faster." These automatic thoughts can cause you to feel upset and angry, and in turn, you will leave the grocery store quickly and may forget some things that you need to buy. Alternatively, the frustration could make you just want to get out of the grocery store as quickly as possible.

Automatic thoughts like these occur all the time in our daily lives, and if they are making us upset, then those accumulated upsetting events can cause us to feel stressed out and even depressed.

Throughout this program, and also in our lives, we will come across situations that will make us upset and will create unpleasant thoughts that in turn make us feel upset or sad. Unfortunately, we cannot avoid unpleasant situations all the time as we are human and we need to go outside of our houses, go to work, and mingle with people.

We need to accept that things will not always turn out the way we would like them to be and that we cannot avoid unpleasant situations. Rather than avoiding them, we must first accept these situations as they appear, observe them, and be present rather than avoiding them. Most of the thoughts come and go from our minds, and we just need to observe them go and don't have to fight them. Remember that most of the thoughts are NOT FACTS.

Let's imagine and discuss a scenario. Imagine you are stuck in traffic for an hour and are upset at yourself, thinking: "I should have left early," "I should have checked the traffic before leaving from the office," "Why did I take this route home instead of taking a different route?" Now imagine the same situation, but this time before you left, your boss called you in his office and told you that you are getting a 50% raise in your salary since you are doing an awesome job, and if you continue to work like that then next year you might be considered for a Vice Presidency situation. Would you be as upset now if you were stuck in traffic? Most likely, you will not be; though the situation is the same, the thoughts are different now. So, remember, our thoughts are not facts. They are just thoughts that sometimes make us upset, but they do pass.

If you continue to have some thoughts that are not going away (e.g., "I am not doing a good job at work," "I will not be able to sleep," etc.), then write down those thoughts in your worry journal. In the evening, process this information and go through the cognitive model to see if that helps you to clarify your thoughts. I am not saying that when you will do the model, your thoughts will go away, but you will have a better idea if your thoughts have any evidence behind them. If they do, then what can you do to solve this worry?

COGNITIVE MODEL:

Situation	Thoughts	Feeling	Evidence for	Evidence against	Most likely/ Alternative
Reached work and feeling tired	I will not be able to work well today.	Frustrated Upset	I am feeling sleepy.	Even when I am tired, it does not affect my work.	I might feel tired today, but it will not affect my work. I might be able to sleep earlier today.

CHAPTER 21

WEEK 3 (CONTINUE TO WORK ON HYPERAROUSAL STATE)

Congratulations on finishing week 2. How did you do? I hope you are progressing well, and I am hoping by the end of this week, you will start sleeping well.

If you are not sleeping better, think about things that are hindering your sleep. Are you sleeping and waking up at the same time? Are you following good Sleep Hygiene? Are you able to decrease your Hyperarousal State?

Please consider walking/exercising in the morning when you wake up. If you cannot spend a lot of time during your morning, then consider walking/exercising even for just 15 minutes.

Try to practice mindful breathing 2-3 times a day for 3-5 minutes.

Remember to write down anything that is bothering you on a piece of paper or on your cellphone, and then you can worry about it during your "Worry Time" in the evening.

Only use the bed for being intimate or for sleep. Remember that the more you will fight to go to sleep, the more difficult it will get to do so; so, if you cannot sleep at night after 15-20 minutes in bed, then get up and do a relaxing activity like reading a book, listening to music, cleaning your wardrobe, etc.

Review your Week 2 Sleep Diary and calculate your Sleep Efficiency. You can write down your Sleep Efficiency by following this chart:

Sleep Efficiency	How much to change my sleep time
84% or less	Go to bed 15 minutes later
85% - 89%	Go to bed at the same time as last week
90%-94%	Go to bed 15 minutes earlier
95% or higher	Go to bed 30 minutes earlier

Keep documenting your Sleep Pattern in the following Sleep Log:

	Mon	Tue	Wed	Thu	Fri	Sat	Sun
Went to Bed							
Fell Asleep							
How many times awake during night							
Total time awake during night							
Wake up time							
Came out from bed							
Total time spend in bed							
Total sleep time							
Sleep Efficiency							

This week, we will also talk about the Gratitude Journal and Progressive Muscle Relaxation. Ideally, you would like to get as many tools as possible in your toolbox to help with your Hyperarousal State.

Gratitude Journal: A gratitude journal is a very simple way to document what we are grateful for in our lives. We often get so busy and worry about the difficulties we face every day that we forget to be grateful for the great things that we have in our lives.

Writing in a gratitude journal lowers your stress level and makes you feel relaxed. When you're feeling down, you can read your gratitude journal, and that can help you get through a difficult day.

So, what do you write in a gratitude journal?

There are many things you can write. Some people write in their gratitude journal every day, some do so 2-3 times a week, and some do it weekly. I would recommend at least writing in it once a week if you cannot do it more frequently. You can write in it in your evening time, and you don't have to spend more than 5-10 minutes each time.

You can write many things, including:

- You are thankful for your partner; why?

- You are grateful for your friend; why?

- You are grateful for the city you live in; why?

- You are grateful for your siblings/parents; why?

- You are thankful for your schoolteacher; why?

- You are grateful for a wonderful day today; why?

- You are thankful for someone who helped you.

- You are happy about three things at work, and what are those things?

- You are proud of yourself for how you managed a difficult situation last week.

- You are grateful for your health, and what are you doing to keep yourself healthy?

PROGRESSIVE MUSCLE RELAXATION:

When we're feeling stressed out, we tend to have parts of our body that tense up. When I get stressed out, I immediately notice tension in my neck and lower back area. If I don't take care of my stress, then I usually have that soreness for a few days. Progressive Muscle Relaxation is a great exercise to get your muscle tension down within minutes. It's better to do this exercise on a regular basis as you will get more benefits from it by doing it on a regular basis compared to doing it only when you are noticing muscle tightness.

In this exercise, you will work on each muscle individually and will keep your focus on the muscle you are working on. You will tense a muscle (not too tense to hurt) and then release that muscle. You will also monitor your breathing during these exercises. If you are having any area in your body in which you have increased pain or injury, talk to your doctor before doing this exercise.

You can do this exercise by sitting or lying down. You can either keep your eyes open or close them.

Breathe in and breathe out. Notice each of your breaths. Breathe normally as you usually do. Feel your breath being cool when you inhale and warm when you exhale. Try to live in the moment, and if you get distracted, then gently bring your attention back to the moment.

You will start with your feet and move up. Gently tense your toes and hold them tightly. Keep your attention on the feeling of tension and keep breathing. You can keep in this tensed state for 5 seconds and then release the tension. Once you release the tension, pause in the feeling of relaxation for 5 seconds.

Now tense your calves for 5 seconds and then release for 5 seconds. Focus all your attention on your calves and feel the tension and the following release of tension as well.

Now you can move to your thighs and tense them. Keep breathing. Keep yourself in the current moment. Feel the tension, keep it tense for 5 seconds, and then release the tension. Have the muscle relax for 5 seconds and then move to your stomach area.

You can do the 5-second tension and 5-second release for the remaining parts of the body, such as your stomach, chest, shoulders, arms, thumbs, fingers, neck, and face.

Once you finish with this exercise, slowly open your eyes. You can also stand up and do some muscle stretching if you like.

CHAPTER 22

WEEK 4 (SLEEP MEDICATIONS)

LIST OF COMMON SLEEP MEDICATIONS:

Sleep medications are intended for use for 4-6 weeks only. Remember that sleep medication will not cure insomnia, It can help temporarily. CBTi is the first-line treatment for chronic insomnia. If CBTi does not work, then a person can have a consultation with their doctor to see if sleep medication can be prescribed for a short duration of time.

Even if you are on medications, you can still benefit from CBTi. You don't necessarily have to stop sleep medication while you are trying a non-medicinal approach to help with your sleep. There are many people who start CBTi treatment while taking medications, and gradually the medications are tapered down by their outpatient provider. Please don't try to stop or taper down your medications on your own, as this can cause problems with your sleep. People also can have withdrawal symptoms if they stop medications abruptly.

I usually recommend that you designate specific days when you will take medications (e.g., Monday and Wednesday), try not to take it more than 2-3 times a week, or only use it when you cannot sleep well for two consecutive nights. Don't take it if you have less than 6 hours to sleep. Again, I recommend for you to discuss the frequency and dosage of taking the medication with your prescriber first.

Sleep medication helps a person go to sleep and/or helps with the maintenance of sleep. It causes suppression of REM sleep and can also suppress deep sleep. As it causes suppression of deep sleep, people sometimes don't feel that their quality of sleep was as good as when they got sleep naturally.

Temazepam (Restoril):

It's a benzodiazepine. These reduce your deep sleep and REM sleep. It can reduce sleep onset, so you can go to sleep early. It also helps with sleep maintenance, so you don't wake up as frequently. Benzodiazepines help with anxiety as well. Benzodiazepines, as a class of medications, can be habit-forming.

Prolonged use of the medication can cause memory problems. It's better that people who are above 65 years of age don't use this medication as it can also cause problems with balance. If you feel tired the next day, don't drive a car or operate heavy machinery as the medication can cause problems with coordination.

Common side effects include fatigue or tiredness the next day. In older populations, it can cause confusion and forgetfulness.

Do not mix this medication with alcohol as it can potentially be very dangerous and can cause respiratory depression.

Dosages range from 7.5 mg to 30 mg at nighttime. It usually takes around 30 minutes to an hour to feel the effects, so it is better to take it around 30 minutes to an hour before bedtime. Be sure once you take this medication that you don't operate any heavy machinery.

If someone has addiction problems (alcohol or any other illicit drug usage problem), that individual should not use this medication as it can be habit-forming.

If you are taking this medication for a long period of time, you cannot stop it abruptly, or you will experience withdrawal symptoms, including rebound insomnia.

Zolpidem (Ambien):

Ambien does bind to a subtype of a benzodiazepine receptor, so although it's not a true benzodiazepine medication, it can still be habit-forming. It's still is not as strong of a habit-forming mediation as benzodiazepines are, though.

Ambien decreases deep sleep and REM sleep, but it does not cause as much of a reduction in that phase as a benzodiazepine might. Regular Ambien helps with sleep onset, and Ambien CR helps with the maintenance of sleep. It can also cause sleepwalking. Some people also will wake up in the middle of the night and will eat from their fridge and will not remember anything occurring. If you start taking this medication, I recommend discussing with your partner/family members that you are starting this medication so they can keep an eye on you to ensure that you don't experience any sleepwalking.

The most common side effect is next-day sleepiness. It's always better to be in bed when you take this medication as it can cause tiredness and, in some people, can cause dizziness.

Elderly patients should avoid taking this medication as it can cause memory problems, and they are also at higher risk of falls.

Zaleplon (Sonata):

Just like Ambien, Zaleplon (Sonata) also binds to a subtype of benzodiazepine receptors, so it can be habit-forming as well. It helps with initiating sleep but usually does not help with sleep maintenance.

Common side effects include tiredness, sleepiness, and dizziness. Elderly populations should avoid the medication due to the high risk of falls.

Eszopiclone (Lunesta):

This helps with sleep onset and sleep maintenance. One of the side effects is a metallic taste, which in some people can be managed by drinking orange or lemon juice. It also binds to a subtype of benzodiazepine receptor, so it can be habit-forming although still not as habit-forming as traditional benzodiazepines (Lorazepam, Clonazepam, Alprazolam).

It can also cause increased sleepiness the next day. Make sure to be in bed or around your bed once you take the medication so when you feel sleepy, you can go to bed.

Suvorexant (Belsomra):

This medication has a unique mode of action: it blocks the action of orexin. Orexin usually helps us keep awake, so when this medication blocks orexin to send wakefulness signals, you start feeling sleepy.

Common side effects include increased tiredness and headache.

It is also habit-forming, so you need to be careful when you take this medication and consider only taking it for a short period of time.

Ramelteon

This medication works by binding to melatonin receptors in order to increase melatonin. It is not a habit-forming medication. Research on medications that increase melatonin or even just taking over-the-counter melatonin supplements has been confusing and unclear.

Doxepin:

This is an older antidepressant called a tricyclic antidepressant (TCA). It works on the serotonin, norepi-nephrine, and histamine receptors. It is FDA-approved to use for patients who have problems with frequent awakening, so it helps with sleep maintenance. The dose range is high if you use it for depression, but for sleep-related uses, the dosing range is low.

The most common side effects of Doxepin include sedation and constipation. In some cases, it can also cause weight gain. Remember that if you are using this medication at a lower dose for sedation, the chances of getting side effects is lower.

OFF-LABEL USAGE OF MEDICATIONS:

Trazodone:

Trazodone is an antidepressant that came into the market as an antidepressant but is now used for sleep-related issues more than for its antidepressant effects.

The good thing about Trazodone is that it does not cause a disturbance in deep sleep. It also does not have the potential for dependence.

Common side effects include nausea, dry mouth, blurry vision, and constipation.

Diphenhydramine (Benadryl):

This is an anti-allergy medication. People can develop sleep tolerance pretty quickly. Caution is recommended in using it in older populations as it can cause confusion.

Seroquel:

Seroquel is an antipsychotic medication. It can cause increased appetite, weight gain, increase blood sugar levels, and elevated liver enzymes, but that does not mean that every individual will have those side effects. If you are using this medication, it's best to have your medical provider order labs to ensure you are not developing any additional medical problems.

Remeron:

Remeron is an antidepressant that has the side effect of sedation, especially in lower doses. It also can cause increased appetite and weight gain.

Melatonin:

There is not a lot of data behind the usage of melatonin for insomnia. Some people with circadian rhythm disorder use it at a low dose. People tend to have a preference for using it since it is more "natural." Some people have even used it in the morning and at night and in varying doses.

DISCONTINUATION OF SLEEP MEDS:

It's never a good idea to decrease any medication or stop any medication without discussing the action with your medical provider. If you abruptly stop a sleep medication, you can go through significant withdrawals, and that can adversely affect your sleep.

If you are on sleep medication and would like to stop taking it, discuss the matter with your care provider. Sometimes tapering down and stopping sleep medication can take a few weeks, but you can do CBTi while going through slow tapering off your medication. Combining CBTi and a gradual taper is very helpful and more likely to be successful.

Tapering down medication can cause rebound insomnia, and there will be nights that you likely will not be sleeping well.

In my experience, it's not a good idea to start CBTi and the tapering of medication at the same time. Let your body get used to CBTi first for a few weeks, and then start tapering down your medications gradually.

CHAPTER 23

WEEK 5 (MOOD PROBLEMS AND SLEEP)

DEPRESSION:

People who suffer from depression have trouble going to sleep, and when they wake up, they don't feel refreshed in the morning. They can also have problems with frequent awakening. On the other hand, if people don't sleep well, they are also more prone to feeling depressed.

Some people with depression feel excessively tired due to their condition and tend to have increased sleepiness, as well as sleeping more during the day and nighttime.

People with depression have a persistent low mood or an irritable mood for most parts of the day. They have feelings of hopelessness and helplessness. They are not enjoying things that they use to enjoy in the past, and their energy levels are very low. They have a hard time focusing on things and also have a hard time with their school studies and tasks at work. Either they don't want to eat, or they want to eat a lot. They can have trouble going to sleep, trouble with waking up a lot, or they can also tend to sleep a lot. They sometimes can also have suicidal thoughts.

If you feel that you are suffering from depression, consider talking to a doctor or counselor. Depression is a treatable illness, but if left untreated, it can affect the quality of a person's life.

When a person is being treated for depression, they will generally notice an improvement in their sleep.

BIPOLAR DISORDER:

People who suffer from bipolar disorder have significant problems with their sleep. If a person suffers from bipolar disorder type 1 and is going through a manic episode, they generally have sleep-related trouble that can last up to a week where they don't feel like sleeping, they have a lot of energy, and their mind is racing. They also can have other symptoms like:

Expansive, elevated, or irritable mood

AND

Three or more of the following symptoms, which must be present and represent a significant change from their usual behavior:

- Inflated self-esteem or grandiosity
- Decreased need for sleep
- Increased talkativeness
- Racing thoughts
- Easily distracted (Their attention is too easily drawn to unimportant or irrelevant external stimuli)
- Increase in goal-related activity or psychomotor disturbance
- Engaging in behaviors that hold the potential for unpleasant consequences (e.g., engaging in unrestrained buying sprees, sexual indiscretions, or foolish business investments)

People who suffer from bipolar disorder type 2 have less intense sleep problems when they are in their hypomanic episodes, but they can still go without sleep for up to four days.

If you or your loved ones suffer from bipolar symptoms, please have yourself or your loved ones evaluated as soon as possible by a health care provider as this is a treatable illness. If left untreated, it can cause significant problems in people's quality of life, social life, family life, and work.

Once bipolar disorder is appropriately treated, the patient's insomnia also typically gets better.

WEEK 6 (IF SLEEP PROBLEMS PERSIST)

Congratulations on finishing five weeks of Sleep Training. I hope by now you are sleeping better. Please continue to follow the basics of this training for the rest of your life. I highly recommend that you try to wake up at the same time most days, if not all days of the week.

Continue to practice meditation as it will not only help you with your sleep but will also help you with obtaining a better quality of life.

Try to exercise regularly and follow good sleep hygiene. There will be days that you will not be able to follow everything you learned during this course, but that is okay.

If you have days that you still don't sleep well, remember that those will pass, and you will start sleeping well again. Don't try to force yourself to sleep if you cannot sleep. If you have a hard time going to sleep, get up out of your bed, do something relaxing, and go to bed once you are feeling sleepy. If you start having thoughts like "I will never be able to sleep well," remember these are just thoughts and NOT facts. Try to be mindful and be in the moment. Do some meditation for 3 minutes and try to focus on the moment.

If your sleep problems still persist after the program, then first analyze if you properly followed everything that we discussed in these pages. Did you go to bed and wake up from bed at the same times? If you didn't follow the Sleep Restriction rules, consider trying again to see if this time you are able to sleep better. If you followed the program well but are still unable to sleep well, consider talking to a sleep specialist to see if they have any suggestions. Your sleep specialist should also make sure that you don't have any additional sleep problems going on, such as sleep apnea. You can also consider talking to your primary care doctor to ensure that you are doing well medically and there is no medical problem causing you to have trouble with sleep.

REFERENCES

American Psychiatric Association. Diagnostic and statistical manual of mental disorders, 5th ed; 2013.

Angarita GA, Emadi N, Hodges S, Morgan PT. Sleep abnormalities associated with alcohol, cannabis, cocaine, and opiate use: a comprehensive review. Addict Sci Clin Pract. 2016 Apr 26;11(1):9. doi: 10.1186/s13722-016-0056-7. PMID: 27117064; PMCID: PMC4845302.

Baglioni C, Battagliese G, Feige B, Spiegelhalder K, Nissen C, Voderholzer U, Lombardo C, Riemann D. Insomnia as a predictor of depression: a meta-analytic evaluation of longitudinal epidemiological studies. J Affect Disord. 2011 Dec;135(1-3):10-9. doi: 10.1016/j.jad.2011.01.011. Epub 2011 Feb 5. PMID: 21300408.

Ballesio A, Aquino MRJV, Kyle SD, Ferlazzo F, Lombardo C. Executive Functions in Insomnia Disorder: A Systematic Review and Exploratory Meta-Analysis. Front Psychol. 2019 Jan 30;10:101. doi: 10.3389/fpsyg.2019.00101. PMID: 30761049; PMCID: PMC6363670.

Beck, J. Cognitive Behavioral Therapy: basics and beyond, 2nd ed. New York: Guilford Press; 2011.

Becker PM. Pharmacologic and nonpharmacologic treatments of insomnia. Neurologic Clinics. 2005 Nov;23(4):1149-1163. DOI: 10.1016/j.ncl.2005.05.002.

Benca RM. Behavioral and pharmacologic management options for insomnia. Postgrad Med. 2004 Dec;116(6 Suppl Insomnia):23-32. doi: 10.3810/pgm.12.2004.suppl38.259. PMID: 19667688.

Driver HS, Taylor SR. Exercise and sleep. Sleep Med Rev. 2000 Aug;4(4):387-402. doi: 10.1053/smrv.2000.0110. PMID: 12531177.

Espie, C. A., Inglis, S. J., Tessier, S., & Harvey, L. (2001). The clinical effectiveness of cognitive behaviour therapy for chronic insomnia: implementation and evaluation of a sleep clinic in general medical practice. *Behaviour research and therapy*, *39*(1), 45–60.

Jackowska M, Brown J, Ronaldson A, Steptoe A. The impact of a brief gratitude intervention on subjective well-being, biology and sleep. J Health Psychol. 2016 Oct;21(10):2207-17. doi: 10.1177/1359105315572455. Epub 2015 Mar 2. PMID: 25736389.

Kabat-Zinn, J. Full catastrophe living: using the wisdom of your body and mind to face stress, pain, and illness. New York: Bantam Dell; 2009.

Ma X, Yue ZQ, Gong ZQ, Zhang H, Duan NY, Shi YT, Wei GX, Li YF. The Effect of Diaphragmatic Breathing on Attention, Negative Affect and Stress in Healthy Adults. Front Psychol. 2017 Jun 6;8:874. doi: 10.3389/fpsyg.2017.00874. PMID: 28626434; PMCID: PMC5455070.

Morin CM, Benca R. Chronic insomnia. Lancet. 2012 Mar 24;379(9821):1129-41. doi: 10.1016/S0140-6736(11)60750-2. Epub 2012 Jan 20. Erratum in: Lancet. 2012 Apr 21;379(9825):1488. PMID: 22265700.

Morin CM, Culbert JP, Schwartz SM. Nonpharmacological interventions for insomnia: a meta-analysis of treatment efficacy. Am J Psychiatry. 1994 Aug;151(8):1172-80. doi: 10.1176/ajp.151.8.1172. PMID: 8037252.

Qaseem A, Kansagara D, Forciea MA, Cooke M, Denberg TD; Clinical Guidelines Committee of the American College of Physicians. Management of Chronic Insomnia Disorder in Adults: A Clinical Practice Guideline From the American College of Physicians. Ann Intern Med. 2016 Jul 19;165(2):125-33. doi: 10.7326/M15-2175. Epub 2016 May 3. PMID: 27136449.

Roehrs T, Roth T. Sleep, sleepiness, sleep disorders and alcohol use and abuse. Sleep Med Rev. 2001 Aug;5(4):287-297. doi: 10.1053/smrv.2001.0162. PMID: 12530993.

Sateia MJ. International classification of sleep disorders-third edition: highlights and modifications. Chest. 2014 Nov;146(5):1387-1394. doi: 10.1378/chest.14-0970. PMID: 25367475.

Spielman AJ, Saskin P, Thorpy MJ. Treatment of chronic insomnia by restriction of time in bed. Sleep. 1987 Feb;10(1):45-56. PMID: 3563247.